MAKE ME A MORNING PERSON

THE
MORNING
PHENOMENON

It Doesn't Take The World To
Get Up Early

BOBBY MARSH

Table of Contents

Chapter 1:

How To Become A Morning Person

Our natural sleep/wake cycles are known as our circadian rhythm, and they can vary a lot from person to person. People fall into different groups, or chronotypes, depending on whether they feel most awake and alert in the morning, in the evening or somewhere in between.

No chronotype is inherently better or worse than another. There's nothing wrong with staying up late and sleeping in. "If that schedule fits with your lifestyle and your obligations, it's not necessary to change it."

The trouble comes when your late bedtime clashes with your early morning obligations. If you're regularly getting less than the recommended seven to nine hours of sleep a night, your health and well-being can suffer.

Unfortunately, we can't pick our chronotypes. Genetics plays a part in whether you identify as a night owl or a morning lark. Still, your habits and behaviours can reinforce those natural tendencies. And those habits aren't set in stone. "By making behavioural changes, you may be able to shift your sleep schedule preferences,"

How to reset your circadian rhythm? How, exactly, do you become more of a morning person?

Shift your bedtime: Count back from the time your alarm rings, aiming for a total of seven to nine hours a night. That will be your target bedtime — eventually. If you're used to turning in well after midnight, willing yourself to suddenly fall asleep at 10:00 p.m. is sure to backfire.

Aim to go to bed 15 or 20 minutes earlier than usual for a few days. Then push it back another 15 minutes for several more days. "It's important to adjust your sleep time gradually," she says.

Make it routine: A quiet bedtime routine is key to helping you fall asleep earlier. At least an hour before lights out, dim the lights and power down your electronics. Find something soothing to do, like taking a warm bath, reading a book or listening to a (not-too-stimulating) podcast. "Give yourself time to wind down and prepare your mind for bed."

Lighten up: "Our circadian rhythms are responsive to light and dark," Exposure to bright light first thing in the morning helps you feel more alert and also helps shift your internal rhythm toward an earlier wake time.

Natural light is the best, so get outside or open your bedroom window. If you can't get outside or your room is natural light-deprived, try a light therapy lamp that mimics the spectrum of natural light.

Make mornings more pleasant: Try to schedule something to look forward to in the morning so that getting up feels like less of a slog. Perhaps a hot cup of coffee, sipped in silence, and the daily crossword puzzle. Knowing that something pleasant awaits can help you take that first, painful step out of bed.

Move your alarm clock: Hitting snooze is all too tempting, so remove that option. Try putting your alarm clock across the room, so you have to get up to turn it off.

Some apps make it even harder to sleep in, by forcing you to engage in mentally stimulating activities like solving a puzzle to stop the beeping. "Do whatever works to keep you from hitting snooze,"

Chapter 2:

9 Habits To Wake Up Early

Waking up early is a real struggle for many people. People are battling this friendly monster silently. Friendly because the temptation to snooze the alarm or turn it off completely when it rings in the morning is irresistible. Almost everyone can attest to cursing under their breath when they hear their alarm go off loudly in the morning.

Here are 9 habits that you should strive to incorporate into your life if you wish to make waking early a part of your routine:

1. Sleeping early.

It is simple – early to bed, early to rise. Retiring to bed early will give you enough time to exhaust your sleep. The average person ought to have at least 8 hours of sleep. Sleeping early will create more time for rest and enable you to wake up on time.

Since sleep is not ignorable, you may be embarrassed when you find yourself sleeping when attending a meeting, or when you are at work. Save yourself this shame by sleeping early to wake up earlier.

After a long day of vicissitudes, gift your body the pleasure of having a good night's rest. Create extra time for this by lying horizontally early enough.

2. Scheduling your plans for the day beforehand.

A good plan is a job half done. Before the day ends, plan for the activities of the next day. When it is all mapped out, you will sleep with a clear mind on what you will be facing the next day. Planning is not a managerial routine task alone but everyone's duty of preparing to fight the unknown the following day.

Waking up early is a difficult decision to make impromptu because of the weakness in yielding to the temptation of 'sleeping for only five more minutes.' Having a plan gives you a reason to wake up early.

3. Creating deadlines.

Working under pressure is an alternative motivation for waking up early if planning has failed. With assignments to submit within a short time, or work reports to be submitted on short notice, the need to wake up early to beat these deadlines will be automatic.

We can create deadlines and ultimatums for ourselves without waiting on our superiors to impose them on us. This self-drive will last longer and it will increase our productivity instead of waiting for our clients and employers to give us ultimatums.

4. Being psychologically prepared.

The mind is the powerhouse of the body. Mental preparedness is the first step towards making and sticking to landmark decisions. The mind should initiate and accept the idea of waking up early before you can comfortably adopt this new routine.

Develop a positive attitude towards rising early and all other subsequent results will fall in place. The first person you need to convince to move towards a particular cause is you. As simple as waking up early seems, many people are grappling with late coming.

This is fixable by making a conscious decision to turn around your sleeping habits. The greatest battle is fought in the mind, where the body antagonizes the spirit.

5.   Finding like-minded friends.

Birds of the same feathers flock together. When you are in the company of friends with one routine, your habits are fortified. With no dissenting voice amongst your friends to discourage you from waking up early, your morning routine will find a permanent spot in your life.

The contrary is true. When you are the odd one out in a clique of friends who have no regard for time, you are likely to lose even the little time-consciousness you had. They will contaminate you with their habits and before you know it, you will slip back to your old self (an over sleeper).

When you also decide to be a loner and not associate with those with the same habits as yourself, then you risk giving up on the way. The psych from friends will be lacking and soon you will just revert to your old habits.

When you want to walk fast, walk alone. When you want to go far, walk with others.

6. Being sensitive to your environment.

It takes a man of understanding to read and understand the prevailing times and seasons. You may occasionally visit a friend or a relative and spend the night. How can you wake up way past sunrise in a foreign environment? This will suggest to your hosts that you are lazy.

Create a good image by waking up a little bit early. If allowed, help do some morning chores over there.

Adjust your routine accordingly. Win over people by waking up early to join them in their morning chores. It is there where friendships are forged. A simple habit of waking up early can be an avenue to make alliances.

7. Addressing any health issues early.

In case of any underlying health conditions that can stop you from waking up early in the morning, seek medical help fast. You may be willing to be an early riser but may be suffering from asthma triggered by the chilly weather in the morning.

When that condition is controlled, you can also manage to wake up a little bit earlier than before and engage in health-friendly activities in the morning. It is a win-win. In either case, going for a medical check-up frequently will keep you healthy to wake up early.

Your health is a priority and when taken care of you will wake up early.

8. It is a habit for the successful.

Ironically, those who have made it in life wake up earlier than the less established ones. One would think that it is the place of the less-founded ones to rise early to go to work and do business so that they can be at par with the wealthy and mighty. Instead, the reverse is true.

Follow the footsteps of great leaders who wake up early to attend to their affairs. They have become who they are because they give no room to the laziness of waking up late. We all have 24 hours in a day to do our businesses, where does the gap between the haves and the have-nots come from? That gap comes from how we use our time.

9. Having a cheerful Spirit.

A cheerful spirit finds joy in even what seems trivial. You should not see waking up early as punishment. It should be a routine to be followed happily religiously. When you have a cheerful spirit, knowing for whose benefit you rise early, then it will be a habit engraved into your spirit.

The above 9 habits to wake up early are key to discovering our purpose and build a new routine henceforth of being an early riser. The most successful people in the world abide by this routine so why not make it yours too.

Chapter 3:

Happy People Plan Their Week in Advance for Maximum Productivity

There you are, enjoying a perfectly beautiful Sunday evening. You've had an eventful and fun weekend and decided to spend tonight chillaxing. Then, from out of nowhere, a sense of dread washes over you (there arose such a clatter?). Your mind begins to think about what you need to get done this week. There's just no way to stop these thoughts once they get rolling.

But, how exactly should you plan your week so that it will be more productive? Well, here are two tips that will guarantee that your week will be efficient and effective.

1. Get a head start

"Sunday clears away the rust of the whole week." — Joseph Addison

It's true. If you want to have a productive week, then you need to start planning on Sundays. If that's not your cup of tea, though, then at least begin your preparations on Friday afternoon or Saturday.

I know. You want to kick back and relax this weekend. But, is it going to be the end of the world if you do a little work? Could you map out your week while watching football or waiting for your favorite HBO to start?

Set aside about an hour and jot down everything you need to get done this week. In particular, think about your daily routines, recurring events, deadlines, and goals. Next, mark them off first so that nothing else gets scheduled ahead of them. Don't forget about anything else that you've penciled in. Remember you are going to that concert with a friend or your family coming to town?

That may sound like a lot of work. But, it gets all of these commitments out of your head. From there, you can begin to plan accordingly. For example, because you have family arriving on Thursday, you'll probably want to make sure that you get your most important work done in advance so that you can spend time with them.

2. Use the E/N/D system.

The E/N/D system, which stands for Energizing / Neutral / Draining, can be used to help you prioritize your time. It accomplishes this by helping you manage your energy.

Whenever scheduling tasks, designate them as either E, N, or D. Usually, energizing tasks are the things you enjoy doing. As such, you would want to schedule them when you need an energy boost, like after lunch. Draining tasks are those that you dread because they're challenging. Those should be scheduled when you have the most energy, like in the morning.

Chapter 4:

How Not To Waste Your 25,000 Mornings As An Adult.

Adulthood is the time of our lives when we need to get serious about everything. We have to take care of every single thing from time to our mornings. Early morning is the time of the day when freshness consumes us—known as the best time to work. Why waste such precious time? Having a good morning automatically means having a good day too. When a mind is fresh, it works. And wasting 25,000 mornings of your adulthood would be truly foolish. Those 3571 weeks would go to waste as there was no essential work done.

To make sure that you don't waste your morning is to be sure that you have mornings. Waking up late just automatically means that half of your day has gone to waste. So, wake up early. Those early hours have some courage to work in them. And who wants to waste such an opportunity to prove themselves. Not only will it be beneficial for your professional life, but it will also be beneficial for your health. Get a decent night's sleep, and you will see the changes that come along with them.

After you open your eyes in the morning, immediately sit up. Going back to sleep is always a more intriguing option. But we need to know that our priority is to wake up. And when you are sleeping, make sure that nothing disturbs it. Phone on silent—the tv's off and lights out. Make sure you are as comfortable as possible so you won't wake up the following day grumpy. Disturbance in sleep may cause the disappearance of it. There is a chance that you can't sleep again. That is not what we want. So, we take things beforehand.

An easy way to wake up in the morning is to have some encouragement ready for you. Either it's gym or work. It will make you wake up in the morning early to jump-start whatever you have planned. Then the mornings will be a lot more efficient for you and much more enjoyable. The first thing that we tend to do right after waking up is to check our phones. We waste 20 minutes or more just lying there doing nothing much of a task. Let's get one thing clear. It's not worth it. Wake up in the morning, get a cup of coffee, and start your day without any technology, naturally.

Once you fall into a habit, you will fall into a routine. Your life will change for the good, and you will look towards the brighter side of life. Mornings are a precious time, and 25,000 of our adulthood is the most important morning of our life. So, make sure that you make every morning out of those 25,000 mornings count. It won't be easy, but it will be worth it!

Chapter 5:

Happy People Have A Morning Ritual

For many of us, mornings begin in a rushed panic. We allow our alarm clocks to buzz at least a dozen times before deciding we have to get out of bed. Then we rush around our homes half-awake, trying to get ready for our day. In a hurry, we stub our toe on the bedpost, forget to put on deodorant, and don't pack a lunch because we simply don't have time. It's no wonder that so many folks despise the thought of being awake before 9 a.m.!

So it may not surprise you to know that the happiest and healthiest people tend to enjoy their mornings. They appear to thrive on waking up with the sun and look forward to a new day of possibilities. These people have humble morning rituals that increase their sense of well-being and give their day purpose.

Here are 3 morning habits that healthy and happy people tend to share:

1. They wake up with a sense of gratitude

Practicing gratitude is associated with a sense of overall happiness and a better mood—so it makes sense that the happiest and healthiest people we know start the day with a gratitude practice. This means that they're truly appreciative of their life and all of its little treasures. They practice small acts of gratitude in the morning by expressing thankfulness to their partner each morning before they rise from bed. They may also write about their gratefulness for five minutes each morning in a journal that they keep by their bedside.

2. They begin every morning anew.

The happiest and healthiest people know that every day is a brand-new day—a chance to start over and do something different. Yesterday may have been a complete failure for them, but today is a new day for success and adventure. Individuals who aren't ruined by one bad day are resilient creatures. Resiliency is a telltale sign of having purpose and happiness.

3. They take part in affirmation, meditation, or prayer.

Many of the happiest folks alive are spiritual. Affirmations are a way of reminding ourselves of all that we have going for us, and they allow us to engrain in our minds the kind of person we wish to be. Meditation helps keep our mind focused, calms our nerves, and supports inner peace. If you're already spiritual, prayer is a great way to connect and give thanks for whatever higher power you believe in.

Chapter 6:

Overcoming Tiredness and Lethargy

Tiredness and lethargy has become a major problem for youths and adults these days. As our lives get busier and our ability to control our sleep gets more out of hand, we all face a constant struggle to stay alert and engaged in our life's work every single day. And this problem hits me as well.

You see, many of us have bad sleep habits, and while it might feel good to stay up late every night to watch Netflix and binge on YouTube and Instagram posts, we pay for it the next day by being a few hours short of a restful night when our alarm wakes us up abruptly every morning.

We tell ourselves that not needing so much sleep is fine for us, but our body tells us a different story. And we can only fake being energetic and awake for so long. Sooner or later we will no doubt experience the inability to function on an optimal level and our productivity and mood will also be affected accordingly. And this would also lead to overall tiredness and lethargy in the long run.

Before we talk about what we can do to counter and fix this problem that we have created for ourselves, we first have to understand why we consciously allow ourselves to become this tired in the first place.

I believe that many of us choose entertainment over sleep every night is because we are in some ways or another overworked to the point that we don't have enough time to ourselves every single day that we choose to sacrifice our sleep time in order to gain back that few hours of quality personal time. After spending a good 10 hours at our jobs from 9-6pm, and after settling down from the commute home and factoring in dinner time, we find ourselves with only a solid 1-2 hours of time to watch our favourite Netflix shows or YouTube, which i believe is not very much time for the average person.

When presented with the choice of sleep versus another episode or two of our guilty pleasure, it becomes painfully obvious which is the "better" choice for us. And we either knowingly or unknowingly choose entertainment and distraction over health.

Basically, I believe the amount of sleep you choose to give yourself is directly proportionate to how happy you are about your job. Because if you can't wait to get up each and everyday to begin your life's work, you will give yourself the best possible sleep you can each night to make sure you are all fired up the next day to crush your work. But conversely, if you hate your job and you feel like you have wasted all your time at work all day, you will ultimately feel that you will need to claim that time back at night to keep yourself sane and to keep yourself in the job no matter how much you dislike it. Even if it means sacrificing precious sleep to get there.

So I believe the real question is not how can we force ourselves to sleep earlier every night to get the 8 hours of sleep that we need in order not to feel tired and lethargic, but rather is there anything we can change about how we view our job and work that we come home at the end of the day feeling recharged and fulfilled to the extend that we don't have to look for a way to escape every night into the world of entertainment just to fill our hearts.

When you have found something you love to do each day, you will have no trouble going to bed at 10pm each night instead of 1 or 2am.

So I challenge each and everyone of you to take a hard look at WHY you are not getting enough sleep. There is a high chance that it could boil down to the reason I have described here today, and maybe a change in careers might be something to consider. But if you believe that this tiredness and lethargy is born out of something medical and genetic, then please do go see a doctor to get a medical solution to it.

Chapter 7:

The Keys To Happiness

If I ask you "what is happiness?", then what would your answer be? It's probably difficult to come up with a simple answer. Yet, here you are, looking for a key to happiness and how to lead a fulfilling life.

The truth is that a universal key to happiness is a myth.

That doesn't mean that you should stop looking for yours right now, it only means that you need to be careful when reading articles about "a key to happiness". The universal key to happiness is non-existent because happiness is one of the most difficult things in life to define.

Now, let's go back to that difficult question: "what is happiness?"

Have you thought about it already? Let me give you an example of how hard it is to define happiness.

Right now, I'm drinking a cup of coffee while writing the outline of this article about how to define happiness. Am I happy right now? Yes, I'm feeling pretty happy:

- I've got nothing to worry about.
- All my basic needs are met.
- The weather is nice.
- I'm going outside in a couple of minutes to go for a walk.

These things are all making me feel pretty happy right now.

By that logic, let's define my happiness as follows:

"Happiness is when I'm in a worry-free state, the weather is nice, everybody I know is alright and I can enjoy a hot cup of coffee."

Voila. There it is. My definition of happiness.

The keys to my happiness are obvious now, and I know enough in order to lead the happiest life I can. I just need to focus on the things I listed above.

Wait a second... If it were this simple, then why have I ever been unhappy?

You might have guessed it already, but I made a very simple error. I assumed that what makes me happy today will make me happy for the rest of my life. And that's just wrong.

Happiness is something that not only changes from person to person, but it's also constantly evolving from day to day.

Your definition of happiness changes over time. This is why happiness is such a difficult concept, and why there's not a single "key to happiness". Whoever tells you otherwise is likely not aware that people change, and that people don't always share the same values, goals, and purposes.

For a minute, I want you to do consider your own happiness. I want you to think back of last week, and consider what things you did that had a positive effect on your happiness.

What things had a significant influence on your mood? What comes to your mind?

Was it spending time with your friends? Was it a great movie you watched? Did you attend an exciting sports event? Or did you enjoy sipping hot coffee on a sunny Wednesday morning? It could obviously be just about anything!

The most important thing to remember when trying to define your keys to a happy and fulfilling life is simple:

There is no universal key that leads to your happiness. That's because your happiness is unique in each and every single way

Chapter 8:

5 Ways To Focus on Creating Positive Actions

Only a positive person can lead a healthy life. Imagine waking up every day feeling like you are ready to face the day's challenges and you are filled with hope about life. That is something an optimist doesn't have to imagine because they already feel it every day. Also, scientifically, it is proven that optimistic people have a lower chance of dying because of a stress-caused disease. Although positive thinking will not magically vanish all your problems, it will make them seem more manageable and somewhat not a big deal.

All you have to do is focus on the positive side of life. It is not necessarily true that people with a positive mindset always get disappointed. Positivity is like a breath of fresh air for us. Looking at the bright side of things has its advantages, and it has its very own benefits. So, positive energy is an essential factor to produce in oneself to make them more efficient in the ways of life. They tend to focus on all the good things and push aside all the wrong things, making them love everything they do.

1. **Think Positively**

Positive thinking is what leads to positive actions, actions that affect you and the people around you. When you think positively, your actions show how positive you are. You can create positive thinking by focusing on the good in life, even if it may feel tiny thing to feel happy about because when you once learn to be satisfied with minor things, you would think that you no longer feel the same amount of stress as before and now you would feel freer. This positive attitude will always find the good in everything, and life would seem much easier than before. You then become the person you once imagined yourself to be, just by thinking positively about it. So, make sure to process those positive thoughts thoroughly for better results or action.

2. Be Grateful

Being grateful for the things you have contributed a lot to your positive behavior. Gratitude has proven to reduce stress and improve self-esteem. Think of the things you are grateful for; for example, if someone gives you good advice, then be thankful to them, for if someone has helped you with something, then be grateful to them, by being grateful about minor things, you feel more optimistic about life, you feel that good things have always been coming to you. Studies show that making down a list of things you are grateful for during hard days helps you survive tough times. Also, be thankful to yourself for making achievements that you wanted. It makes you feel positive about yourself and makes your confidence boost through you. You have to make sure that you know what it is to be thankful for. Be grateful to someone for all the right reasons, and you will feel positive.

3. Laugh Through Situations

A person laughing always looks like a happy person. Studies have shown that laughter lowers stress, anxiety, and depression. Open yourself up to humor, permit yourself to laugh even if forced because even a forced laugh can improve your mood. Laughter lightens the mood and makes problems seem more manageable. Your laughter is contagious, and it may even enhance the perspective of the people around us. Smiling is free therapy. You have to pass an approving smile and make someone's day up.

4. Don't Blame Yourself For The Things You Can't Control

People with depression or anxiety are always their jailers; being harsh on themselves will only cause pain, negativity, and insecurity. So try to be soft with yourself, give yourself a positive talk regularly; it has proven to affect a person's actions. A positive word to yourself can influence your ability to regulate your feelings and thoughts. The positivity you carry in your brain is expressed through your actions, and who doesn't loves an optimistic person. Instead of blaming yourself, you can think differently, like "I will do better next time" or "I can fix this." Being optimistic about the complicated situation can lead your brain to find a solution to that problem.

5. Start Your Day with A dose of Positivity

When you wake up, it is good to do something positive in the morning, which mentally freshens you. You can start the day by reading a positive quote about life and understand the meaning of that quote, and you may feel an overwhelming feeling after letting the meaning set. Everybody loves a good song, so start by listening to a piece of music that gives you positive vibes, that gives you hope, and motivation for the day. You can also share your positivity by being nice to someone or doing something nice for someone; you will find that you feel thrilled and positive by making someone else happy.

Conclusion

Indeed, we can not just start thinking positively overnight, but we have to push ourselves more every time to improve. Surround yourself with brightness, good people, and a positive mindset—a good combination for a good life.

Chapter 9:

6 Ways To Adopt A Better Lifestyle For Long-Term Success

A good lifestyle leads to a good life. The important choices we make throughout our lives impact our future in numerous ways. The need to make ourselves better in every aspect of life and the primary ability to perform such a routine can be a lifestyle. There is no proper way to live written in a book; however, through our shared knowledge and our comprehension, we can shape a lifestyle that can be beneficial and exciting at the same time. Though there is no doubt that falling into a specific routine can be difficult but, maintaining a proper state is more critical for a successful life.

For long-term success, a good lifestyle is a priority. Almost everything we do in our lives directly or indirectly involves our future self. So, a man needs to become habitual of such things that can profit him in every way possible. To visualize a better you, You need to configure just about everything around you. And to change all the habits that may make you feel lagging. The most common feature of a better lifestyle for long-term success is determination.

1. Change In Pattern Of Your Life

It is good to shape a pattern of living from the start and forming good habits, engaging yourself in profitable practice, and choosing a healthier custom. It feels impossible to change something you have already been habitual of, but willpower is the key. With some motivation and dedication, you can change yourself into a better version of yourself. You are choosing what might be suitable for you and staying determined on that thought. The first step is to let go of harmful things slowly because letting go of habits and patterns that you are used to can be challenging. After some, sometime you will notice yourself letting go of things more easily.

2. Take Your Time

Time is an essential factor when it comes to forming a lifestyle for a successful life. Time can seem to slow through the process, making us think that it may have been stopped in our most difficult moments. Similarly, making us feel it goes flying by when our life is relaxed and at ease. Time never stops for anyone. It is crucial to make sure we make most of our time and consume it in gaining more knowledge and power. Take time to inform your lifestyle, but not more than required. We are taking things at a moderate pace so you can both enjoy life and do work.

3. Don't Always Expect Things To Go Your Way

As much as we humans like to get our hopes high, we can't always expect things to go our way. Even things we have worked hard for can sometimes go downhill. It is at times overconfidence, but sometimes it can be pure bad luck. We can't get disheartened by something that was not meant to go a specific way. Don't expect perfection in all the work you do. Staying patient is the walk towards the reward. And making the best out of the worst can be the only way to get yourself going.

4. Don't Be Afraid To Ask For Help

It is human nature to ask each other for help now and then. If it comes to this point, don't be afraid to ask for help yourself. Ask someone superior to aid you on matters you find difficult. Don't hesitate to ask your inferiors who might have more knowledge than you in some certain customs. Help them, too, if needed. Ask them to assist you out on points, but never make them do the whole project. Don't make someone do something you wouldn't do yourself.

5. Be Prompt In Everything

Lagging behind your work can be the worst possible habit you could raise. Make yourself punctual in every aspect. Make sure you are on time everywhere. Either it's to wake up in the morning or to go to a meeting. Laziness can never be proven good for you or your dream towards a prosperous lifestyle. Respect time, and it shall respect you. Show your colleges that they can depend on you to show up on time and take responsibility for work. You would rather wait than making others wait for you. That will show you seriousness toward your business.

6. Keep A Positive Attitude

Keeping a positive attitude can lead to a positive lifestyle. Be happy with yourself in every context, and make sure that everything you do has your complete confidence. Be thankful to all who surround you. Keep a positive attitude, whether it be a home or office. Speak with your superiors with respect and make yourself approachable around inferiors. Your positive mindset can affect others in a way too. They will become more inclined towards you, and they can easily suggest you help someone.

Conclusion

Just about everything in your life affects your future in a way or other, so make sure that you do all you can to make yourself worth the praise. Keep your lifestyle simple but effective. Try to do as much as possible for yourself and make time to relax as well. For long-term success, willpower is the most important; make sure you have it. Keep your headlight and calm for the upcoming difficulties and prepare yourself to face almost everything life throws at you.

Chapter 10:

Happy People Stay Present

"Realize deeply that the present moment is all you ever have."

According to a study, 50% of the time, we are not fully present in the moment. We are either thinking about the past or worrying about the future. These things lead to frustration, anxiety, and pain in our daily life. Each morning as soon as we wake up, we start seeking distractions. As we wake up with a clear mind, we should be grateful for a new day that we got; instead, we start looking for our phone, start going through interwebs and rush into our days. So now we are going to help you and list some of the things that will help you stay present.

Stop Being a Slave to Your Mind: For the next four days, let's do an exercise where you pay attention to your thoughts and see what crosses your mind. You. You will soon realize that majority of the thoughts that you have are destructive. There will be very little time to think about the present, and the majority of your thoughts would be about the past or the future. So, whenever this happens and you find yourself wandering consciously, try to bring yourself back to the present. Also, you need to remind yourself that multi-tasking is a myth and focus on one thing only.

Tap into Your Senses: If you mindfully tap into your senses, you will realize that it is a fantastic way of bringing more awareness into your day. Because our eyes are wide open all day, we can see, but we forget to tap into other senses such as taste, touch, or smell. But if you use these, you can feel more present and calm down if you are in a stressful situation. You might not realize this, but our senses play a huge role in manifesting our reality. For example, everything we are hearing we are touching will regularly turn into our reality. That is why we can use the power our senses have and feel more calm and present.

Listen Closely: Everyone loves to talk, but only a few people like to listen. People love to share their dreams, what they have accomplished and what they desire, and still, nobody seems to be listening closely.

"When you talk, you are only repeating what you already know. But if you listen, you may learn something new."

When you listen carefully, you will be able to charm people and at the same time learn new things and be present. Because you will be focusing on what they are saying, you will focus on the current moment. This way, you will also be able to silence your thoughts about the past and future because you will be consciously listening and focusing on what they are saying. This will also benefit your relationship in the long run because when you need an ear to listen to your problems, they will be there for you. This is a win-win situation for you, and you will improve your relationship while practising being more present.

Chapter 11:

To Make Big Gains, Avoid Tiny Losses

Life is a process of adding and subtracting. We add the things that make us better and make life easier. We put aside the things that prove to be a pebble in the shoe.

There is a flaw in human effort and our concept for success. We think that we can achieve more if we focus harder on getting better. We think that if we are not getting worse, we are on the right track. But I can assure you, we are heavily mistaken.

The more we focus on bigger gains, the more we overlook the small things we stop caring about. We give up on relations, hobbies, ethics, love, and the million other losses that we don't measure on the same scale.

We can achieve the same amount of things, the same scale of success, and still, be the better person that we want to be. But we don't need to not work on the smaller details of this successful journey.

Let's say you have achieved it all and now you look back a decade or two. Do you think you won't regret the things that could have been saved in this whole process? But you chose not to or didn't care enough for them, and now you are rich in the pocket but poor in every other sense.

They say money can buy you anything, but it can never buy you happiness. You can have all the money in the world but you can't make sure if you won't ever have any regret.

We all are a creator. We make things, sometimes for ourselves and sometimes for people around us. Sometimes we make things better for us that then prove to be good for someone else as well. But also do things in a way that doesn't affect anyone else in a bad way. At least not deliberately.

Bad things happen, but most of the time we are the reason for them to happen in the first place. We are so devoted to the greater good that we neglect the small things we lose in the process.

Check it with yourself, if you are so devoted to being a better person than you were yesterday, and you have achieved more than yesterday. Then why do you still repeat the small mistakes and take the small losses?

You have to understand the concept of losses over gains. If you invest some money into something, and you are at a small loss every other day, then you can't justify the big profits you might gain some days later.

It is the constant concern to keep away from the small misfortunes or mistakes that might leave you into yet another breakdown. If you truly want to be a free and successful person, you need to have confidence in whatever you do will certainly give you more and more and it won't come at the cost of a single thing.

Take the mantra, reduce your losses and your gains will gain volumes in no time.

Chapter 12:

Get Your Brain To Focus On What Matters

The very first step r the very first feeling close to success is that you are capable of visualizing it every day and every night. If your brain is so focused on what matters and has a much clearer vision of the final product of your efforts, then you have the best friend you could ever wish to see.

If your brain can do this, you have done the biggest and most difficult task of your life, that is, training your brain to think of things just as your will dictates you.

We live in an era of technology so reliable yet also disturbingly manipulative that we cannot think of a single thing more important than our phone if we lose one.

Think about it, You wake up on the alarm of your phone. You snooze it and you check your feed. You check IGN, Twitter, and other social media platforms to check if someone approached you or if something more havoc has occurred anywhere on the planet. We are always so dependant on the technology around us that we cannot take an hour out of this ecosystem to make something more meaningful with our time.

We are often told that we have a limited time on this planet and there are a lot more things to achieve in life. But what do we do to make things seem more meaningful than what we do on our phones?

So what to do in such an era of technology to be more productive?

I would say, stop keeping your phone in your pocket. I can assure you this idea is not as stupid as it may sound initially. But hear me for a second.

We have a different screen for a different environment. We use an IPad or a Tablet when we want to relax on a couch for Netflix. We use our laptops for office work strictly. We use a desktop for gaming and stuff. But our phones, we carry everywhere.

We wake up with it and we sleep with it. We cannot commute without it, which I know is justified but we don't commute all day long. So why do you need to keep it in your pocket for the rest of the day?

Start this practice today for a better chance. Use a traditional alarm clock over your phone. When you want to read the news over breakfast, use a newspaper. When you are in the office, put your phone on your desk and switch it to the meeting.

Life has a lot of important things for you to do. You need to take some time out of everything you do for yourself in a day and devote some of it to your friends family and your other half.

How much more time do you need for yourself, when you sleep a third of your day just so you can function properly the next day. So start thinking of new ways to use your time for making more money rather than sulking over others' success just by looking at some social media post.

Chapter 13:

Happy People Do What Matters to Them

Think about what you want most out of life. What were you created for? What is your mission in life? What is your passion? You were put on this earth for a reason, and knowing that reason will help you determine your priorities.

I spent a total of four months in the hospital, healing from my sickness. During that time, I spent a lot of time thinking about my purpose in life. I discovered that my purpose is to help you change your lives by focusing on what matters most to you.

1. Create A Plan

Create a plan to get from where you are today to where you want to be. Maybe you need a new job. Maybe you need to go back to school. Maybe you need to deal with some relationship issues. Whatever it is, create a plan that will get you to where you want to be.

While I was in the hospital, I began to draft my life plan. My plan guides all of my actions, helps me focus on my relationships with my wife and daughter, and helps me keep working toward my life purpose. A life plan will help you focus your life too.

2. Focus On Now

Stop multitasking and focus on one thing at a time. It may be a project at work. It may be a conversation with your best friend. It may just be the book that you have wanted to read for months. The key is to focus on one thing at a time.

I plan each day the night before by picking the three most important tasks from my to-do list. In the morning, I focus on each one of these tasks individually until they are completed. Once I complete these three tasks, I check email, return phone calls, etc.

3. Just Say "No."

We all have too much to do and too little time. The only way you will find the time for the things that matter is to say "no" to the things that don't.

I use my purpose and life plan to make decisions about the projects and tasks I say yes to. If a project or task is not aligned with my purpose, a good fit with my life plan, and sometimes that I have time to accomplish, I say no to the project. Saying no to good opportunities gives you time to focus on the best opportunities.

Research tells us that 97 percent of people are living their life by default and not by design. They don't know where their life is headed and don't plan what they want to accomplish in life.

These steps will help you to decide what matters most to you. They will help you to begin living your life by design and not by default. Most importantly, they will help you to create a life focused on what matters to you.

Let me end by asking, "What matters most to you?

Chapter 14:

The Easiest Way to Live a Short, Unimportant Life

An essential and successful life may seem intriguing but, sometimes it's just a lot of work. Whereas, in comparison, a short and unimportant life seems easier to live. The one reason for this may be that you need to eat up your surroundings. People who donate to this world live longer. So, you don't donate. You consume the world. But there is no doubt that people who live longer have many advantages, whereas someone living a short life would not have time for that. Not only is it a loss, but it will affect your life in which you are breathing already.

Few things can lead a person to an unimportant and unhealthy lifestyle. Of course, no one can control how many days we will live on this planet but, we can contribute to our surroundings. And even if you come up with small things, they can impact your life somehow. Be yourself when it comes to shaping. Don't let this world shape you but yourself. It may not only change your life but, it can also give them the confidence to others to change their lives.

It would help if you believed that you could live. If you give up on your life, life will give up on you. Keep yourself worth running in every factor of life. It would be best if you made yourself feel worth it to keep up with the world. Live a meaningful life by all means. How? By contributing to things, talk with a friend, take a long walk in the mornings, or call the people you care about. Even saying hi to a stranger count as contributing to this world. And small contribution leads towards a more significant source of the outcome.

Talk with yourself about how you are going to live this life, and live, not survive. Thet both are different things. We won't know if tomorrow will be our last day, so we got to live it today as it is. Nowadays, we tend to live our lives by ourselves. We prefer to talk on the phone instead of meeting up. It just leads towards an unhealthy and unimportant life. Meet up if you can. Contribute your ideas or decisions to that plan. Make sure that you work out your best if you want it to be done.

A short and unimportant life may seem easier to live by but, it's non-enjoyable. It's full of disadvantages and losses from every side. Isn't it better to live? To give it all your best? We need to devote most of ourselves to this one life that we got. And live each day to its fullest.

Chapter 15:

The 5 Second Rule

Today I'm going to share with you a very special rule in life that has worked wonders for me ever since I discovered it. And that is known as the 5 second rule by Mel Robbins.

You see, on a daily basis, I struggle with motivation and getting things done. I struggle with the littlest things like replying an email, to responding to a work request. This struggle has become such a bad habit that before I think about beginning any sort of work, I would first turn on my Netflix account to watch an episode or two of my favourite sitcom, telling myself that I will get right on it after I satisfy this side of me first.

This habit of procrastination soon became so severe that I would actually sit and end up wasting 4-5 hours of time every morning before I would actually even begin on any work-related stuff. Before I knew it, it would be 3pm and I haven't gotten a single thing done. All the while I was staring at the clock, counting the number of hours I have wasted, while simultaneously addicted to procrastinating that I just could not for the life of me get myself off the couch onto my desk to begin any meaningful work.

I realized that something had to change. If I kept this up, I would not only not get anything done, like ever, but i would also begin to loathe myself for being so incredibly unproductive and useless. This process of self-loathing got worse everyday I leaned into the habit of procrastination. It was only until i stumbled onto Mel Robbin's 5 second rule that I started to see a real change in my habits.

The rule is simple, to count backwards from 5 and to just get up and go do that thing. It sounded stupid to me at first, but it worked. Instead of laying around in bed every morning checking my phone before I woke up, I would count backwards from 5 and as soon as it hit 1, i would get up and head straight towards the shower, or I would pack up my things and get out of my house.

I had identified that staying at home was the one factor that made me the most unproductive person on the planet, and that the only way I knew I was going to get real work done, was to get out of the house. I had also identified that showering was a good way to cleanse my mind from the night before. I really enjoyed showering as I always seem to have a clear head afterwards to be able to focus. What works for me, may not necessarily work for you. You have to identify for yourself when are the times you are most productive, and simply replicate it. A good way to find out is by journaling, which I will talk about in a separate video. Journaling is a good way to capture a moment in time and a particular state of mind. Try it for yourself the next time you are incredibly focused, write down how you got to that state, and simply do it again the next time to get there.

The 5 second rule is so simple yet so powerful because it snaps our unhealthy thought patterns. As Mel puts it, our brain is hardwired to protect us. We procrastinate out of fear of doing the things that are hard, so we have to beat our brain to it by disrupting it first. When we decide to move and take action after reaching 1, it is too late for our brains to stop us. And we get the ball rolling.

I was at my most productive on days that I felt my worst. But I overcame it because I didn't let my brain stop me from myself. I wouldn't say that I am struggle free now, but i knew i had a tool that would work most of the time to get me out of procrastination and into doing some serious work that would move my life forward. There are times when I would forget about the 5 second rule and my bad habits would kick in, but I always reminded myself that it was available to me if I chose to use it.

I would urge all of you who are struggling with any form of procrastination or laziness to give the 5 second rule a try. All you need to do is to get started and the rest becomes easy.

Chapter 16:

The Daily Routine Experts for Peak Productivity

What is the one thing we want to get done for a successful life? That is an effective daily routine to go through the day, every day. History is presented as an example that every high achiever has had a good routine for their day. Some simple changes in our life can change the outcome drastically. We have to take the experts' advice for a good lifestyle. We have to choose everything, from color to college, ourselves. But an expert's advice gives us confidence in our choice.

You have to set the bar high so that you get your product at the end of the day. Experts got their peak productivity by shaping their routine in such a way that it satisfies them. The productivity expert Tim Ferriss gave us a piece of simple yet effective advice for such an outcome. He taught us the importance of controlling oneself and how essential it is to provide yourself with a non-reactive practice. When you know how to control yourself, life gets more manageable, as it gives you the power to prevent many things. It reduces stress which gets your productivity out.

Another productive expert of ours, Cal Newport, gives us his share of information. He is always advising people to push themselves to their limits. He got successful by giving his deep work more priority than other work. He is managing multitasks at the same time while being a husband and a father. He is a true example of a good routine that leads to positive productivity. It would help if you decided what matters to you the most and need to focus on that. Get your priorities straight and work toward those goals. Construct your goals and have a clear idea of what your next step will be. It will result in increasing your confidence.

Now, the questions linger that how to start your day? Early is the answer. Early to bed and early to rising has been the motto of productive people. As Dan Ariely said, there is a must 3 hours in our day when our productivity is at its peak. A morning person hit more products, as it's said that sunrise is when you get active. Mostly from 8 o'clock to 10 o'clock. It's said that morning is the time when our minds work the sharpest. It provides you alertness and good memory ability. It is also called the "protected time." We get a new sense to think from, and then we get a sound vision of our steps and ideas to a routine of peak productivity.

Charles Duhigg is a known news reporter, works for the New York Times. He tells us to stop procrastinating and visualizing our next step in life. Not only does it give you confidence, but it also gives you a satisfactory feeling. You get an idea of the result, and you tend to do things more that way. This way, you get habitual of thinking about your next step beforehand. Habits are gradually formed. They are difficult to change but easy to assemble. A single practice can bring various elements from it. Those elements can help you learn the routine of an expert.

You will eventually fall into place. No one can change themselves in one day. Hard work is the key to any outcome. Productivity is the result of many factors but, an excellent daily routine is an integral part of it which we all need to follow. Once you fall into working constantly, you won't notice how productive you have become. It becomes a habit. There might be tough decisions along the way, which is typical for an average life. We need to focus on what's in front of us and start with giving attention to one single task on top of your priority list. That way, you can achieve more in less time. These are some factors and advice to start a daily routine for reaching the peak of productivity with the help of some great products.

Chapter 17:

6 Tricks To Become More Aware Of Your Strengths

"Strength and growth come only through continuous effort and struggle." - Napoleon Hill.

While it is true that we tend to focus more on our weaknesses than on our strengths, it is also true that we should polish our strengths more than our weaknesses. This in no way means that we should consider ourselves superior to others and start looking away from that we have flaws. Unfortunately, most of us don't spend much time on self-reflection and self-awareness. But they are the vital aspects if we are thinking of improving ourselves in any way.

Here are 6 Tricks to become more aware of your strengths:

1. Decide to be more self-aware

Human beings are complicated creatures. Our minds are designed so that we tend to absorb more negative than positive thoughts about ourselves and others. For this reason, self-awareness is perhaps the most crucial thing in an individual's life. Self-awareness is the ability to look deep inside of yourself and monitor your emotions and reactions. It is the ability to allow yourself to be aware of your strengths, weaknesses, as well as your triggers, motivators, and other characteristics. We'll help you find a set of tricks and techniques that you can apply to polish your strengths in a self-awareness way; and how to use your strengths in a promising way.

2. Meditation:

The first thought that will come to your mind would be, "Is this person crazy? How can meditation help us improve our strengths?" But hear me out. The fresh breeze of the morning when everything is at peace, and you sit there inhaling all the good energy in and the bad energy out, your mind and thoughts would automatically become slow-paced and calm. Once you get to relax with yourself, you can analyze the things that have been happening in your life and develop possible solutions on how you can deal with them using your strengths. The positive energy and calming mood you will get after meditating would help you make your decisions wisely when you are under pressure and your mind is in chaos.

3. Labelling your thoughts:

More often, our thoughts reflect on our behavior and what makes us fail or succeed in life. People can genuinely relate to a situation where they could have possibly thought about a worst-case scenario, but in the end, nothing as such happened. Our anxiety and hopelessness don't come from the situation we are struggling with, but rather our thoughts make us believe in the worst possible things that could happen to us. But we're stronger than we give ourselves credit for. We have the power to control our negative thoughts and turn them into positive ones. We can list all the ideas and thinking that provide us with stress and tension and then label them as either useful or useless. If the particular thought is causing a significant effect in your life, you can work towards it to make your life better and less anxious. Know your priorities and take help from your strengths to tackle the problems.

4. **Befriending your fears:**

There's not a single person on this planet who isn't afraid of something. Be it the fear of losing your loved ones or any phobias of either animal, insects, heights, closed spaces, etc. There are also so many fears related to our self-worth and whether we are good enough, skilled enough, or deserving enough of anything. To accept these fears and work towards overcoming them is perhaps the most powerful thing one could do. It takes so much of a person's strength and willpower to befriend fear, reduce it, and finally eliminate it. Most of the time, we end up in situations that we always feared, and then we have to take quick actions and make wise decisions. To remain calm in such cases and use your strengths and experiences to tackle whatever's in front of you is a remarkable quality found in only a few. But we can also achieve and polish this quality by strengthening our minds and preparing ourselves to get us out of situations wisely and effectively. To be patient and look into the problems from every angle is the critical component of this one.

5. **Watching your own movie:**

Narrating your life experiences to yourself or a close friend and telling yourself and them how far you have come can boost your self-confidence immensely. You should go in flashbacks and try to remember all the details of your life. You will find that there were some moments you felt immense joy and some moments where you felt like giving up. But with all the strength that you were collecting along the way, you endured the possible tortures and struggles and challenges and eventually rose again. So you should focus and be well aware of how you tackle those situations, what powers you have, and the strengths that couldn't let you give up but face everything. Once you have found the answers to the above questions, like for example, it was your patience and bravery that helped you through it, or it was your wise and speedy decisions that made it all effective, you can understand what strengths you have and make use of them later in life too.

6. Motivate yourself:

We should stop looking for others to notice how great we did or stop waiting for a round of applause or a pat on the back from them. Instead, we should motivate ourselves every time we fall apart, and we should have the energy to pick ourselves back up again. The feeling of satisfaction we get after completing a task or helping someone, that feeling is what we should strive for. We should become proud of ourselves and our strengths, as well as our weaknesses, that they helped us transform into the person we are today. We should never feel either superior or inferior to others. Everyone has their own pace and their own struggles. Our strengths should not only be for ourselves but for others too. Kindness, empathy, hospitality, being there for people, patience, courage, respect are all the qualities that one must turn into their strengths.

Conclusion:

The key to perfection is self-awareness. There's a fine line between who you are and who you strive to become; it can be achieved by becoming aware of your strengths, polishing them, and creating a sense of professional as well as personal development. Your strengths motivate you to try new things, achieve new skills, become a better version of yourself. Your strengths are what keeps you positive, motivated, help you to maintain your stress better, aid you in your intuitive decision making, and command you to help others as well. It inspires you to become a better person.

Chapter 18:

5 Tips for A More Creative Brain

Nearly all great ideas follow a similar creative process, and this article explains how this process works. Understanding this is important because creative thinking is one of the most useful skills you can possess. Nearly every problem you face in work and life can benefit from creative solutions, lateral thinking, and innovative ideas.

Anyone can learn to be creative by using these five steps. That's not to say being creative is easy. Uncovering your creative genius requires courage and tons of practice. However, this five-step approach should help demystify the creative process and illuminate the path to more innovative thinking.

To explain how this process works, let me tell you a short story.

A Problem in Need of a Creative Solution

In the 1870s, newspapers, and printers faced a very specific and very costly problem. Photography was a new and exciting medium at the time. Readers wanted to see more pictures, but nobody could figure out how to print images quickly and cheaply.

For example, if a newspaper wanted to print an image in the 1870s, they had to commission an engraver to etch a copy of the photograph onto a steel plate by hand. These plates were used to press the image onto the page, but they often broke after a few uses. This process of photoengraving, you can imagine, was remarkably time-consuming and expensive.

The man who invented a solution to this problem was named Frederic Eugene Ives. He became a trailblazer in the field of photography and held over 70 patents by the end of his career. His story of creativity and innovation, which I will share now, is a useful case study for understanding the five key steps of the creative process.

A Flash of Insight

Ives got his start as a printer's apprentice in Ithaca, New York. After two years of learning the ins and outs of the printing process, he began managing the photographic laboratory at nearby Cornell University. He spent the rest of the decade experimenting with new photography techniques and learning about cameras, printers, and optics.

In 1881, Ives had a flash of insight regarding a better printing technique.

"While operating my photo stereotypes process in Ithaca, I studied the problem of the halftone process," Ives said. "I went to bed one night in a state of brain fog over the problem, and the instant I woke in the morning saw before me, apparently projected on the ceiling, the completely worked out process and equipment in operation."

Ives quickly translated his vision into reality and patented his printing approach in 1881. He spent the remainder of the decade improving upon it. By 1885, he had developed a simplified process that delivered even better results. As it came to be known, the Ives Process reduced the cost of printing images by 15x and remained the standard printing technique for the next 80 years.

Alright, now let's discuss what lessons we can learn from Ives about the creative process.

The 5 Stages of the Creative Process

In 1940, an advertising executive named James Webb Young published a short guide titled, A Technique for Producing Ideas. In this guide, he made a simple but profound statement about generating creative ideas.

According to Young, innovative ideas happen when you develop new combinations of old elements. In other words, creative thinking is not about generating something new from a blank slate but rather about taking what is already present and combining those bits and pieces in a way that has not been done previously.

Most importantly, generating new combinations hinges upon your ability to see the relationships between concepts. If you can form a new link between two old ideas, you have done something creative.

Young believed this process of creative connection always occurred in five steps.

1. **Gather new material.** At first, you learn. During this stage, you focus on 1) learning specific material directly related to your task and 2) learning general material by becoming fascinated with a wide range of concepts.

2. **Thoroughly work over the materials in your mind.** During this stage, you examine what you have learned by looking at the facts from different angles and experimenting with fitting various ideas together.

3. **Step away from the problem.** Next, you put the problem completely out of your mind and do something else that excites you and energizes you.

4. **Let your idea return to you.** At some point, but only after you stop thinking about it will your idea come back to you with a flash of insight and renewed energy.

5. **Shape and develop your idea based on feedback.** For any idea to succeed, you must release it out into the world, submit it to criticism, and adapt it as needed.

Chapter 19:

5 Ways Quitting Something Can Bring You Joy

Do you ever wonder if you will ever be truly happy in your life? Do you wonder if happiness is just a hoax and success is an illusion? Do you feel like they don't exist? I know a friend who felt like this a little while ago. At the time, she was making a six-figure income, was working for her dream company (Apple), and had a flexible work schedule. Despite all this, she was miserable. She would have never been able to quit my job if not for the practice she got from quitting little things.

Of all the things that she tried, quitting these seven little things made her the happiest.

1. Quit Reading the News

News headlines are usually about happenings around the world. Most times, they are negative. Negative headlines make for better stories than positive headlines. Would you read a headline that says 'Electric Chair Makes a Comeback' or a headline that says 'Legislation debate in Tennessee'? See what I mean.

Journalists have to write stories that interest us. I can't blame them for that. Changing the time that I caught up on the news helped me be more positive during the day. Start reading inspirational posts first thing in the morning instead of news. You can still catch the news later, around 11 am instead of at 6 am.

2. Quit Hunching Your Shoulders

This boosted my confidence levels.

We hunch our shoulders and take up as little space as possible when we feel nervous and not too comfortable. This is body language 101.

Keeping a posture, opening up your shoulders will make you feel more confident during the day. But, I must admit it will make you more tired than usual. It will take you at least a total of 45 days before you start doing this effortlessly.

3. Quit Keeping a Corporate Face at Work

We are all trained not to show real feelings at work. Having a corporate face is good for corporate, not for you. Smiling all day, even when you are upset, will lift your mood. It will make you feel better sooner. Studies have shown that smiling makes you happy.

4. Quit Writing Huge Goals

It is better to write and work towards achievable goals before starting to write our stretch goals. Stretch goals are great to push ourselves. But, we all need achievable goals to boost confidence and to have successes that we can build momentum on. This can be hard for you if you are an overachiever.

5. Quit Eating Fries and Eat Oranges Instead

Fries are comfort food for a lot of people. But eating them saps energy.

Eat oranges instead of fries every time you feel down and feel the need for comfort food. This not only boosts your energy but will also help you lose some pounds if you want to. Plus, this will give you energy and clarity of mind.

Chapter 20:

Five Habits That Make You Age Faster

We will all get old one day. A day is coming when we will not have the youthful energy we presently enjoy. Everyone desires that this day should never come or rather come very late in our lifetime. Nevertheless, it is an inevitable occurrence. We can only delay it.

Here are five habits that make you age faster:

1. Unforgiveness

Unforgiveness is like hiding fire expecting that no one will notice. Eventually, the smoke will give you away. It arises when one deeply wrongs us leaving a trail of hurt and agony that cannot easily be forgotten. The offended party will never forget what was committed against him/her. Anytime he/she sees the other person, the bad memory is re-kindled.

It is unhealthy to hold on to such bad memories. They cause mental and emotional trauma. They cause and affect your health. When your health is affected due to your unforgiveness, you bear full consequences and can only blame yourself. However subtle it may seem, unforgiveness is responsible for the fast aging of many people who harbor it.

The offender could probably have even forgotten about it and moved on with his/her life. The victim is the one who will be left bearing the brunt of the hurt. Stress will manifest on your face in the form of contortions making you appear aged than you are. Choose forgiveness always and you will lead a happier youthful life.

2. Bitterness

Bitterness is an aftermath of unforgiveness. It is a very strong emotion that succeeds unforgiveness. Regardless that it springs forth from within, bitterness manifests on the face over time. The glory on the face of a joyous person is absent on that of a bitter person.

Ever asked yourself how people can judge someone's age bracket? The youthful glamour disappears on the face of a bitter person. Some elderly people appear very youthful. The reason is that they live a bitter-free life. Such a type of lifestyle guarantees youthfulness.

Strive to be youthful and live a fulfilling life by keeping bitterness at bay. Entertaining it will increase the rate at which you age and may succumb to old-age diseases while still at a very young age.

3. Lack of Physical Exercise

Physical exercise is an important part of the human routine. It is not reserved for sports people only but everyone needs it to grow healthy. So important is exercise that it is incorporated in the education curriculum for students to observe.

Physical exercises help one become healthy and look youthful. It burns excess calories in our body and unblocks blood vessels thus increasing the efficiency of blood flow and body metabolism. Excess water, salts, and toxins are expelled from our bodies when we sweat after intense exercise.

The lack of physical exercise makes our bodies stiff and they become a fertile ground for lifestyle diseases like high blood pressure. Conversely, exercises improve our body shape and sizes by shedding extra weight. This healthy lifestyle brought by regular exercises will enable us to live a long healthy disease-free life.

4.   Poor Dieting

Dieting serves several purposes but the chief benefit of a proper dieting habit is that it gives the body important nutrients and shields it from excesses caused by human bias. Proper dieting will make you eat nutritive food that you may even not like. The benefits of nutritive meals outweigh your tastes and preferences.

Poor dieting is taking meals without considering their nutritive value or repetitively eating a meal because you love it. This habit makes you caution less with what you eat. You will ingest excess oily and fatty foods which will harm the healthy bacteria that live in your gut. It goes further to affect your heart health and immune response to diseases.

These factors directly affect the rate at which you age. Greasy foods will manifest in your skin and alter your appearance. It may also cause acne on your face. To reduce your aging rate, improve your dieting habit and supply the body with the right nutrients.

5.   Lack Of A Skincare Routine

As much as the skin is affected by the type of meals we take, a healthy skin care routine plays a major role in maintaining youthful skin. There are many celebrities globally who look younger than their age and this has a lot to do with their skincare routine.

It varies from one person to another but the fundamentals are constant - washing your face with plenty of clean water in the morning and evening. This is to remove dirt and dead cells from the skin. When one does not take care of his/her skin, aging creeps in. The face is the most visible part of the human body and it requires maximum care.

Failure to have an efficient skincare routine will entertain old age - the last item on our wish list.

Since we are now enlightened about habits that will make us age faster, the onus is on us to fight them and remain youthful.

Chapter 21:

<u>Why You've Come Too Far To Quit</u>

Remember the first day of school, when someone bullied you for being too nerdy, or for being too whiny. What did you feel when some called you a Four-eye for wearing glasses? What did you do then? How did you answer them? You didn't! Right? Why?

Because you weren't strong enough then to tackle anyone. Because you didn't have any experience to tell you what to do next.

But your parents told you to stop crying and keep doing your thing and one day, everything will be secondary. So you kept your line, didn't indulge in anything anyone else said and you got through that time.

This is the definition of life. Life is a sequence of events that bully you at every corner. But you cannot give up on life, because someone put a dent on your new car or if someone spilled coffee on your shirt.

Things happen because life happens, and you live your life for the things you want to achieve one day.

You dream because you hope for a better future, and that future is worth living for if you have suffered and felt the pain.

Nothing in this life is easy, but nothing is impossible. It may not be possible for you but at the same moment it might be happening for someone else in the world

You have come this far, to achieve the goals your set. You can't give up now only because you haven't seen it yet.

You breathe every day because you have to. Your success has the same needs! You need to give life everything that you got. Not on some days, but every day because it is not something you do when you feel like it, but you have to because you have to live on your terms. No one can dictate your life but only you.

When you feel like quitting, remember why you started it all. You started it to prove everyone wrong. You started it to shun your haters. You started to bully the bullies.

When you feel like quitting, remember, you have too much to fight for and very little to quit for.

When you get up in the morning, remember what you dreamt of last night. Remember your failures and give yourself a chance to prove yourself wrong.

Quitting is for those who are still the kid they were back then. Quitting is for those who still have the feeling that everything will get better on its own - It never does, and it never will. Only if you quit the quitting attitude and start taking initiative for your ultimate dream.

The best you can be is by the best effort you put into being the protagonist of your story. Become the writer of your story. If you want your story to remain average, remain the same person you were a day before.

If your heart tells you to quit, rev up your heart to do one pick one more step towards your penultimate goal. Dictate your heart how bad do you want it.

If you are still the kid who still thinks that things will happen no matter what I do, believe me, you are wrong. This whole attitude of not trying hard enough to achieve your goals is the biggest thing wrong with an average human. But you are not an average human.

The average human wouldn't have the guts to pursue the dream in the first place. An average human wouldn't dream big in the first place. An average human would have given up on the first setback of life and went down a deep hole, only to avoid the problems. But it never is the solution to anything.

Build the guts to keep going no matter what happens. Life will beat you up at every interval. You might have a big setback after every brief moment of happiness.

You might lose friends, family, and everyone you ever cared for. People who were once standing shoulder to shoulder with you might not even care to say your name if they think you don't need what you are striving for. But they don't have a say in your future. It's you who has everything to care for. Everything to account for. So don't give up only because everyone else gave up on you. You are still alive and trying.

Give yourself every chance, to win. Give your life every chance for it to matter. Avail every stone to keep the bullies away, but not by mirroring the act, but your efforts for your goal and they will bow down one day.

Chapter 22:

How To Succeed In Life

"You can't climb the ladder of success with your hands in your pocket."

Every day that you're living, make a habit of making the most out of it. Make a habit of winning today. Don't dwell on the past, don't worry about the future. You just have to make sure that you're winning today. Move a little forward every day; take a little step every day. And when you're giving your fruitful efforts, you're making sure you're achieving your day, then you start to built confidence within yourselves. Confidence is when you close your eyes at night and see a vision, a dream, a goal, and you believe that you're going to achieve it. When you're doing things, when you're productive the whole day, then that long journey will become short in a matter of time.

Make yourself a power list for each day. Take a sheet of paper, write Monday on top of it and then write five critical, productive, actionable tasks that you're going to do that day. After doing the task, cross it off. Repeat the process every day of every week of every month till you get closer to achieving your goals, your dreams. It doesn't matter if you're doing the same tasks every day or how minor or major they are; what matters is that it's creating momentum in things that you've believed you couldn't do. And as soon as the momentum gets completed, you start to believe that you can do something. You eventually stop writing your tasks down because now they've become your new habits. You need a reminder for them. You don't need to cross them off because you're going to do them. The power list helps you win the day. You're stepping out of your comfort zone, doing something that looks uncomfortable for starters, but while doing this, even for a year, you will see yourself standing five years from where you're standing today.

Decide, commit, act, succeed, repeat. If you want to be an inspiration to others, a motivator to others, impact others somehow, you have to self-evaluate certain perceptions and think that'll help you change the way you see yourself and the world. Perseverance, hard-working, and consistency would be the keywords if one were to achieve success in life. You just have to keep yourself focused on your ultimate goal. You will fall a hundred times. There's always stumbling on the way. But if you have the skill, the power, the instinct to get yourself back up every time you fall, and to dig yourself out of the whole, then no one can stop you. You have to control the situation, Don't ever let the situation control you. You're living life exactly as it should be. If you don't like what you're living in, then consider changing the aspects. The person you are right now versus the person you want to be in the future, there's only a fine line between the two that you have to come face-to-face with.

Your creativity is at most powerful the moment you open your eyes and start your day. That's when you get the opportunity to steer your emotions and thoughts in the direction that you want them to go, not the other way around. Every failure is a step closer to success. We won't succeed on the first try, and we will never have it perfect by trying it only once. But we can master the art of not giving up. We dare to take risks. If we never fail, we never get the chance of getting something we never had. We can never taste the fruits of success without falling. The difference between successful people and those who aren't successful is the point of giving up.

Success isn't about perfection. Instead, it's about getting out of bed each day, clearing the dust off you, and thinking like a champion, a winner, going on about your day, being productive, and making the most out of it. Remember that the mind controls your body; your body doesn't hold your mind. You have to make yourself mentally tough to overcome the fears and challenges that come in the way of your goals. As soon as you get up in the morning, start thinking about anything or anyone that you're grateful for. Your focus should be on making yourself feel good and confident enough to get yourself through the day.

The negative emotions that we experience, like pain or rejection, or frustration, cannot always make our lives miserable. Instead, we can consider them as our most incredible friends that'll drive us to success. When people succeed, they tend to party. When they fail, they tend to ponder. And the pondering helps us get the most victories in our lives. You're here, into another day, still breathing fine, that means you got another chance, to better yourself, to be able to right your wrongs. Everyone has a more significant potential than the roles they put themselves in.

Trust yourself always. Trust your instinct—no matter what or how anyone thinks. You're perfectly capable of doing things your way. Even if they go wrong, you always learn something from them. Don't ever listen to the naysayers. You've probably heard a million times that you can't do this and you can't do that, or it's never even been done before. So what? So what if no one has ever done it before. That's more of the reason for you to do it since you'll become the first person to do it. Change that 'You can't' into 'Yes, I definitely can.' Muhammad Ali, one of the greatest boxers to walk on the face of this planet, was once asked, 'how many sit-ups do you do?' to which he replied, 'I don't count my sit-ups. I only start counting when it starts hurting. When I feel pain, that's when I start counting because that's when it really counts.' So we get a wonderful lesson to work tirelessly and shamelessly if we were to achieve our dreams. Dr. Arnold Schwarzenegger beautifully summed up life's successes in 6 simple rules; Trust yourself, Break some rules, Don't be afraid to fail, Ignore the naysayers, Work like hell, And give something back.

Chapter 23:

HOW TO STOP JUDGING YOUR OWN WORK

Have you been extra nice to yourself lately? If you're a writer … the answer is probably: "…mayyyybe?"

Writers — creators in general — are way too hard on themselves. We like making things, and we feel good doing it. But we really want to feel like we're doing a good job.

When we don't feel that way — which happens much more often than we realize — we start to doubt if writing is even worth the struggle.

Why are we so judgmental of our own work? Because it's the easiest to judge. It comes from us. We know it better than anyone.

But we can all learn to be critical without being so harsh. Here's how.

Remind yourself that not everything you write is going to feel polished. And the simple reason for that? The majority of the time, it won't be.

You have to make messes to make masterpieces. You have to do things wrong, you have to not do your best if you're ever going to learn what you're actually capable of. If what you're writing seems terrible — well, it might be. That doesn't mean it always will be, or that it will be the best thing you'll ever write.

You're going to write sentences you're unsure of, paragraphs that just don't "sound quite right." You're going to question whether or not this scene should stay or go. You're going to ask yourself a million times if you're doing any of this right.

What matters most is that you keep writing anyway. You can't polish something unfinished. Even if a draft feels like the worst thing you've ever written, at least you have something to work with — something you can improve little by little until it meets your personal standards (if that's even possible …).

Focus on how you feel about your work, not on how others might react. We're all guilty of imagining how our future readers will react to certain parts of our stories. Sometimes, it's what keeps you going when you're starting to feel unsure. When you laugh at your own writing (admit it — it happens to you too), you picture others laughing too.

But there's a dark side to this train of thought. If we focus too much on what people might think about our writing, we can begin to worry that they won't like it. That they'll tell everyone else not to read it. That our words aren't actually good … that they never will be.

The best way to judge whether or not your writing is meaningful and readable is if it feels that way to you. Yes, your readers matter whether they exist yet or not. You are writing for their entertainment. But until you get your words in front of eyes, the only opinion that matters is yours.

Your inner critic will never stop talking, but you can tune it out. Here's the truth not every writing expert will tell you: you will never stop doubting or judging yourself or your writing. There is no magic cure for self-criticism. But that doesn't mean you can't tone it down enough to avoid letting it interfere with your work.

We judge ourselves more harshly than everyone else does (even though it sometimes feels the other way around) because we genuinely want to do a good job. And deep down we know we are the only ones in control of whether or not we do the work "well."

The problem is, we're so used to seeing others' work and the kinds of writing that gets high praise that we often can't help but compare our drafts to their published masterpieces. When we do that, our writing just never feels "as good." We immediately spiral into "i'll never be good enough" self-talk. We get sad. We stop writing.

That negative self-talk will always be there. You will always hear it.

But you don't have to listen to it.

You don't have to care about the lies it's telling you. You don't have to let them stop you from doing the work you know you're meant to do.

It's one thing to say you're not going to pay attention to your voice of doubt and another to actually ignore it. It's not that simple for a lot of people — and that's ok. Some have an easier time quieting their minds than others. As a writer, it's often one of those things you learn to do the longer you do it, the more you practice it.

That voice in your head telling you that you'll never achieve your dreams? The best thing you can do to demote its scream to a whisper is to prove it wrong.

Chapter 24:

How To Focus on Creating Positive Actions

Only a positive person can lead a healthy life. Imagine waking up every day feeling like you are ready to face the day's challenges and you are filled with hope about life. That is something an optimist doesn't have to imagine because they already feel it every day. Also, scientifically, it is proven that optimistic people have a lower chance of dying because of a stress-caused disease. Although positive thinking will not magically vanish all your problems, it will make them seem more manageable and somewhat not a big deal.

Positive thinking is what leads to positive actions, actions that affect you and the people around you. When you think positively, your actions show how positive you are. You can create positive thinking by focusing on the good in life, even if it may feel tiny thing to feel happy about because when you once learn to be satisfied with minor things, you would think that you no longer feel the same amount of stress as before and now you would feel freer. This positive attitude will always find the good in everything, and life would seem much easier than before.

Being grateful for the things you have contributed a lot to your positive behavior. Gratitude has proven to reduce stress and improve self-esteem. Think of the things you are grateful for; for example, if someone gives you good advice, then be thankful to them, for if someone has helped you with something, then be grateful to them, by being grateful about minor things, you feel more optimistic about life, you feel that good things have always been coming to you. Studies show that making down a list of things you are grateful for during hard days helps you survive through the tough times.

A person laughing always looks like a happy person. Studies have shown that laughter lowers stress, anxiety, and depression. Open yourself up to humor, permit yourself to laugh even if forced because even a forced laugh can improve your mood. Laughter lightens the mood and makes problems seem more manageable. Your laughter is contagious, and it may even enhance the perspective of the people around us.

People with depression or anxiety are always their jailers; being harsh on themselves will only cause pain, negativity, and insecurity. So try to be soft with yourself, give yourself a positive talk regularly; it has proven to affect a person's actions. A positive word to yourself can influence your ability to regulate your feelings and thoughts. The positivity you carry in your brain is expressed through your actions, and who doesn't loves an optimistic person. Instead of blaming yourself, you can think differently, like "I will do better next time" or "I can fix this." Being optimistic about the complicated situation can lead your brain to find a solution to that problem.

When you wake up, it is good to do something positive in the morning, which mentally freshens you up. You can start the day by reading a positive quote about life and understand the meaning of that quote, and you may feel an overwhelming feeling after letting the meaning set. Everybody loves a good song, so start by listening to a piece of music that gives you positive vibes, that gives you hope, and motivation for the day. You can also share your positivity by being nice to someone or doing something nice for someone; you will find that you feel thrilled and positive by making someone else happy.

Surely you can't just start thinking positively in a night, but you can learn to approach things and people with a positive outlook with some practice.

Chapter 25:

10 Habits of Amancio Ortega Gaona

Names like Warren Buffet and Bill Gates are household names, but do you know Amancio Ortega? Amancio is indeed one of the world's wealthiest fashion mogul. He founded Inditex, which is best known for Zara fashion and other men's and women's retail clothing, footwear, and home textiles businesses.

He is regarded as a pioneer in fast fashion thanks to his investment's eye. Zara's fashions are inspired by fashion show looks but are priced affordably to the average person. How did he get to where he is now? Here are 10 habits of Amancio Ortega.

1. Speed Is Entirely Everything

Ortega's "fast fashion" strategy demonstrates that speed is all you need to be ahead of your competitors and gain a market advantage. According to a business insider, a dress shown during Fashion Week can be found in Zara a few weeks later, while the same takes months to be displayed at a department store. His market aggressiveness is scheduled to design new clothes faster than anyone else in the market.

2. Good Things Comes With Patience

Although ten years may seem interminable when starting a business, it pays off. Being patient allows you to wait, observe, and decide when it is appropriate to act. It was after Zara went international 10 years later after trying different business approaches that Ortega broke through. Accordingly, all you need to do is take a step back, regroup, and look for better solutions.

3. It is About What Customers Want

Ortega's fashion sense stems from his observation of what people wear and listening to what they want. As his guiding business model, he does not base his inventory on runway shows but rather on what customers want. The customer must remain your primary focus, both in developing your new designs and the related activities.

4. Introverts Are Also Entrepreneurs

Many successful entrepreneurs, such as Ortega, are not extroverts, as might be expected in their line of work. Ortega once stated that even if you aren't the party's life, you can still run a successful business. He is the type of person who avoids speaking to the press at all costs, so little is known about him.

5. Be Modest and Humble

Ortega's journey is a classic rags-to-riches story, but he has remained true to his humble beginnings. He dropped out of school to start making money. According to The Telegraph, he has never had an office because he prefers working very close with his employees. A humble beginning does not preclude you from becoming successful, and success does not preclude you from remaining modest and humble. Those qualities can be extremely beneficial in both your personal and professional life.

6. Keep On Innovating

As Ortega puts it, "the worst thing you can do is becoming self-satisfied." Success is never guaranteed, so don't be satisfied with what you've already done. If you want to innovate, don't be concerned more with the outcome than the process.

7. Maintain Control Over Supply Chain

When you focus on a specific supply chain, you will undoubtedly respond to new trends accordingly. While many fashion companies stock clothing made in China due to low labor costs, Inditex sources most of its products from Spain, Portugal, and Morocco, according to The Economist in 2012. Ortega's stores only sell what customers want, so there are no unsold items.

8. Keep in Mind What Motivates You

Remembering what makes you wake up early in the morning to do what you do is your drive for success. Take, for instance, Ortega's childhood; he witnessed his mother being denied credit at a grocery store when he was young. At this moment, he was motivated to start working right away so that his family wouldn't have to be in such a situation again.

9. Age Is Not a Limit to Success

Sometimes you're led to believe that you must be successful at a young age, much like Steve Jobs or Mark Zuckerberg. However, Ortega founded Zara when he was nearly 40 years old. While that isn't particularly old by most people's standards, it isn't your typical twenty- or thirty-something millionaire story. It's reassuring to know that it's never too late to pursue your dreams and ambitions, as Ortega did.

10. Enjoy the Finer Things in Life

Despite his modesty and humbleness, Ortega also engages in some fun activities. He spends his free time horse riding and owns a horse riding center in Finisterre, Spain. He also owns a high-end Audi A8 sedan. It's okay to have time for yourself; spend money vacationing if you can afford it.

Conclusion

Amancio Ortega Gaona's success story is truly inspiring, as he rose from nothing to become one of Europe's richest businessmen and fashion pioneers. No matter small you start, you'll surely reach there. But only if you're motivated enough to see it.

Chapter 26:

10 Habits Of Happy People

Happiness is a state of joy. In happiness, one is thrilled, contented, and tickled by joy. It is often expressed through bursts of laughter amidst smiles and it cannot be hidden. Happiness is a state everyone desires but few can maintain. Here are ten habits of happy people:

1. They Are Outgoing

Happy people are very social. They easily interact with strangers and make friends faster than ordinary people. They are charming to a fault and you cannot help but love their company.

Happy people are easily noticeable in a room full of different people. They are conspicuously outgoing to initiate trips, vacations, and team-building activities. Their social nature makes them thrive both in outdoor and indoor interactions.

2. They Are Self-Driven

Happy people have a strong personality that drives them in life. They are not coerced to do something and often act out of self-will. They stand out from a population that requires much convincing before they act.

They live a purposeful life that is crystal in their minds. Happy people do not need an external influence to be happy. They genuinely derive pleasure from what they do.

3. They Wake Up Early

Happy people know the secret of waking up early and do not need persuasion to wake up earlier than everybody else.

In waking up early, they keep off conflict with other people who could ruin their day. They build the foundation of the day ahead of them in the morning and they can maintain the tempo until the end. Strangers can do very little to ruin their happiness.

4. They Are Positive About Life

Happy people are very optimistic about life. Positivity is their middle name. They hardly entertain thoughts of failure. Like all of us, happiness is a choice they have to constantly make and work towards it. It distinguishes them from everyone else.

How can you be happy if you do not see the good out of the ugly? Happy people look at the brighter side of life because the grass is not greener on the other side but where you water it.

5. They Keep The Company Of Other Happy People

Happy people keep the fire of happiness burning because they associate with like-minded people. They share ideas and strategies on how to pursue their purpose. They also encourage each other when hope is bleak.

The company of sad and angry people is devastating because it gives no room for happiness to thrive. Happy people embrace each other's company because it is all they have got if they are to stay happy.

6. They Read Success Stories

Success stories are inspiring. They make us pull our socks and give us hope to succeed as others have. Happy people read and share success stories because therein lies happiness. They bask in the glory of their friends because they believe their turn too shall come.

Happy people shun bad news and stories of despair because they are discouraging and one could succumb to depression if they are not careful.

7. They Know How To Handle Bad News And Rejection

Happy people know that rejection does not spell doom for them. They have hope that they can rise above all challenges they face and still be happy. Unlike ordinary people who take rejection personally and despair, happy people consider it as another phase of life.

Handling bad news is a skill that happy people have perfected. Although some bad news could hit them hard, they know how to soak in their happiness and not live in sadness.

8. They Are Agents Of Change

Happy people are agents of change wherever they go. They make a difference with their speech and their aura changes everything. Everybody can feel the impact of happy people wherever they are.

Happy people inspire others to be like them. They recruit others in their league of happiness because they desire to see a changing world.

9. They Are Loving And Caring

Happy people can afford to be caring because they have no traces of bitterness or anger within them. They genuinely care for the welfare of other people.

Happiness makes people loving unlike those who harbor anger. You can only give what you have and it is natural for happy people to care more and sad people hurt more.

10. They Live An Authentic Lifestyle

Authenticity is a mark of happy people. They live a genuine lifestyle without seeking to impress anyone. Their joy does not lie in the approval of strangers but the satisfaction of their needs.

Happy people live within their financial means and not in the standards that other people have put for them. Their priorities are independent of external influence.

In conclusion, happy people are easy to spot. It is everybody's dream to be happy but a very elusive one. These ten habits of happy people distinguish them from others.

Chapter 27:

9 Habits of Highly Successful People

Success comes to people who deserve it. I bet you have heard this statement quite a few times, right? So, what does it mean exactly? Does it mean that you are either born worthy or unworthy of success? Absolutely not. Everyone is born worthy, but the one thing that makes some people successful is their winning habits and their commitment to these habits.

Today, we will learn how to master ten simple habits and behaviors that will help you become successful.

1. Be an Avid Learner

If you didn't know, almost all of the most successful people in the world are avid learners. So, do not shy away from opportunities when it comes to learning. Wake up each day and look forward to learning new things, and in no time, I bet you will experience how enriching it really is. Also, learning new things has the effect of revitalizing a person. So, if you want to have more knowledge to kickstart your journey in the right direction, here are some things that you can do - make sure to read, even if it is just a page or two, daily. It could be anything that interests you. I personally love reading self-help books. If you are not that much of a reader, you can even listen to a podcast, watch an informative video, or sign up for a course. Choose what piques your interest, and just dive into it!

2. Failure is the Pillar of Success

Most people are afraid to delve into something new, start a new chapter of their lives, and chase after their dreams – all because they are scared to fail. If you are one of those people who are scared to fail, well, don't be! Because what failure actually does is prepares you to achieve your dream. It just makes sure that you are able to handle the success when you finally have it. So when you accept that failure is an inevitable part of your journey, you will be able to plan the right course of action to tackle it instead of just being too scared to move forward. Successful people are never scared of failure; They just turn it around by seeing it as an opportunity to learn.

3. Get Up Early

I bet you have heard this a couple of thousand times already! But whoever told you so was not lying. Almost all successful individuals are early risers! They say that starting the morning right ensures a fruitful day ahead. It is true! Think about it, on the day you get up early, you feel a boost of productivity as compared to when you wake up late and have to struggle against the clock. You will have plenty of time and a good mood to go through the rest of the day which will give you better outcomes. All you have to do is set up a bedtime reminder. This is going to make sure that you enough rest to get up in the morning instead of snoozing your alarm on repeat! Not a morning person? Don't worry. I have got you covered! Start slow and set the alarm 15 minutes before when you usually wake up. It doesn't sound like much, eh? But trust me, you will be motivated to wake up earlier when you see how much difference 15 minutes can make to your day.

4. Have Your Own Morning Ritual

Morning rituals are the most common habit among achievers. It will pump you up to go through the day with a bang! You just have to make a routine for yourself and make sure to follow it every day. You can take inspiration from the morning routines of people you look up to but remember it has to benefit you. So you might be wondering, *What do I include in the ritual?* I would suggest you make your bed first thing in the morning. This might not sound as great a deal, but hey, it is a tested and approved method to boost your productivity. It is even implemented in the military. Doing this will motivate you as you get a sense of achievement as you have completed a task as soon as you woke up. After that, it could be anything that will encourage you, such as a walk, a workout session, reading, journaling, or meditating.

5. Stop Procrastinating

From delaying one task to not keeping up with your deadlines, procrastination becomes a deadly habit. It becomes almost unstoppable! Did you know, most people fail to achieve their dreams even if they have the potential just because of procrastination? Well, they do. And you might not want to become one of them. They say, "Old habits die hard," true, but they do die if you want them to. Procrastination has to be the hardest thing we have to deal with, even though we hey created it in the first place. Trust me, I speak from experience!

So what do you do to stop this? Break your task into small bite-sized pieces. Sometimes, it is just the heaviness of the task that keeps us from doing it. Take breaks in between to keep yourself motivated.

Another thing that you can do is the "minute rule." Divide your tasks by how much time they take. The tasks that take less than 5 minutes, you do it right then. Then you can bigger tasks into small time frames and complete them. Make sure you do not get too lost in the breaks, though!

6. Set Goals

I cannot even begin to tell you how effective goal setting is. A goal gives you the right direction and motivation. It also gives you a sense of urgency to do a task that is going to just take your productivity level from 0 to 10 in no time!

So how do you set goals? Simple. Think about the goals you want to achieve and write them down. But make sure that you set realistic goals. If you find it difficult, don't worry. Start small and slow. Start by making a to-do list for the day. You will find out soo that the satisfaction in ticking those off your list is unbelievable. It will also drive you to tick more of them off!

7. Make Your Health a Priority

Health is Wealth. Yes, it is a fact! When you give your body the right things and make it a priority, it gives you back by keeping you and your mind healthy. I bet you've heard the saying "You are what you eat," and by "eat," it does not simply mean to chew and swallow! It also means that you need to feed your body, soul, and mind with things you want them to be like. Read, listen, learn, and eat healthy. You could set a goal to eat clean for the week. Or workout at least for 10 minutes. And see for yourself how it gives you the energy to smash those goals you've been holding off! Also, great news – you can have cheat days once a week!

8. Plan Your Day the Night Before

"When you fail to plan, you plan to fail." People who succeed in life are not by mere coincidence or luck. It is the result of detailed, focused planning. So, you need to start planning your way to success too. Before you sleep tonight, ask yourself, *What is the most important thing that I have to do tomorrow?* Plan what assignments, meetings, or classes you have to complete. Planning ahead will not only make you organized and ready, it also highly increases your chances to succeed. So, don't forget to plan your day tonight!

9. Master the Habit Loop

Behavioral expert, BJ Fogg, explains that habits are formed around three elements: Cue, Routine, and Reward. Cue is the initial desire that motivates your behavior. Routine is the action you take. And the reward is the pleasure you gain after completion. So why am I telling you all of this? Because this habit loop is how we are wired. It is what motivates us. We seek pleasure and avoid pain. And you can use this loop to your advantage! Let's say you want to finish an assignment. Think of the reason why you want to. Maybe you don't want to fall behind someone or want to impress someone. It could be anything! Now time for you to set your rewards. It could be eating a slice of cheesecake or watching an episode of your favorite series after you've finished. Rewards motivate you when you slack off. Play around until you find a combination that works best for you. You will also need a cue; it could be anything like a notification on your phone, an email, or simply your desire. You can set a cue yourself by creating a reminder.

Habits are what make a man. I hope you follow these habits and start your journey the right way to becoming successful in life.

Chapter 28:

20 Positive Affirmations For Men

A positive affirmation is a statement about yourself that is phrased in the positive, present tense. It reflects an area of your life, emotions, or belief system that you want to improve or change. The potential benefits of affirmations are vast. Positive affirmations empower you to become the best version of yourself. They inspire you to act in ways that help you fulfill your potential. You can use positive affirmations to reprogram negative thoughts into positive beliefs. The ability to reprogram your beliefs about yourself has the potential to transform your life completely.

For an affirmation to be effective, it needs to meet four criteria.

Each positive affirmation you use should be:

1. **Worded in the present tense**
2. **Positive**
3. **Specific**
4. **Personal**

You can create your own positive affirmations using this four-step framework. The benefits of affirmations are dramatically increased when you have created it yourself from an existing negative belief. Let's say you had a belief that you are unsuccessful in your job.

Where focus goes, energy flows. If you keep feeding this belief, it will manifest as truth.

When you understand this, you can see how our thoughts really do shape our reality.Instead, you can use this belief as an opportunity to grow. Take that statement and switch it to its positive opposite. Rather than thinking: 'I am terrible at my job, I'll never get a promotion, my boss hates me,' you now think 'I am great at my job, I love what I do, and I always put 100% effort into every task

Whether you choose to formulate your own positive affirmations or use the ones I have created for you below, you must cultivate a daily practice. The best times to practice are first thing in the morning and last thing at night (or whenever you feel that you need to repeat them to start feeling better). During these times, your mind is more open and will absorb the statements on a deeper level.

It is best if you say them out loud while looking in the mirror. Speaking them to yourself affirms that you trust in yourself, and you believe the statements to be true. If speaking them out loud is not possible, you can say them in your mind. Writing them out a few times a week is also beneficial. Try getting a journal specifically for this purpose. Another technique that you might find useful is to pin the written affirmations to the mirror or refrigerator, where you will see them often.

When you are just beginning with this practice, it may be easy to forget, so set an alert on your phone or in your calendar to remind you. Here are 20 examples of positive affirmations relating to different areas of life.

Choose the ones that resonate most with you.Once you feel that you have integrated those particular statements, you can select or create new ones for other areas you want to improve.

Confidence and Self-Esteem

1: "I feel confident in every situation."

2: "I like who I am."

3: "I am a good person."

4: "I am great at helping people."

5: "I feel valued by my friends and family."

Inner Strength and Resilience

1: "I meet each new challenge with enthusiasm."

2: "I am strong and stable."

3: "I think I can, so I can."

4: "No matter what happens, I can handle it."

5: "I am powerful."

Positivity and Joy

1: **"I radiate joy to everyone I meet."**

2: **"I see the best in people."**

3: **"In the present moment there are no issues, only peace."**

4: **"Happiness is a choice; today, I choose to be happy."**

5: **"I have the power to turn negative thoughts into positive beliefs."**

Career and Success

1: **"I deserve success."**

2: **"I can succeed at whatever I choose."**

3: **"I am good at my job, and I love what I do."**

4: **"I have great ideas."**

5: **"I am innovative and tenacious."**

I hope that my guide to positive affirmations for men has provided you with a solid foundation for designing your perfect practice. Remember, to reap the benefits of affirmations, you should say them out loud every day and write them out a few times a week. Use any of my examples of positive affirmations, or for extra power, try creating your own using my framework. If you commit to a daily practice, you will soon notice the benefits in your career, relationships, emotional resilience, sense of self-worth, and confidence.

Chapter 29:

6 Habits of Oprah Winfrey

When anyone utters the name "Oprah Winfrey," one of her most iconic quotes comes to mind: "You get a car, and everyone else gets a car." While most business people applaud the "to-do roster," Oprah is not one of them; instead, she values meditation, no alarms, and limiting business operations to the necessary minimum. From a poor rural Mississippi upbringing to getting a full scholarship and to landing a seat on the morning talk program, Baltimore Is Talking, to now solidifying her reputation as a global legend and America's first black billionaire, with a net worth of US$2.5 billion, you might be wondering – exactly how she does it?

Oprah Winfrey maintains a series of daily routines-from getting up early to work out to practicing Gratitude. This daily routine, as she notes, keeps her happy, grounded, and humble.

Here are six daily habits from the legend herself that you might want to make your own.

1. Her Day Starts With Morning Rituals.

Oprah Winfrey starts her mornings with a sequence of spiritual exercises, allowing her body to wake up and her mind to focus on Gratitude and self-reflection. She meditates for approximately 20 minutes. If the weather is nice, she sits in her lawn chair with her eyes closed, simply reminiscing on the previous day and imagining her aspirations for the day ahead. She noted that starting the day slowly allows her mind to wake up and become entirely focused on the day ahead.

2. Working Out Every Morning.

Oprah's journey to weight loss has been a struggle over the years. She opened up on her efforts with maintaining a healthy weight and fitness program. She highlighted in an interview that she loves sweating it up through the regular old-fashioned cardio exercises, explicitly on an elliptical machine followed by a treadmill. She then follows with some regular bodyweight training before warming up for some sit-ups.

Although there is ongoing research on whether a better fitness routine should be in the morning or the evening, substantial studies describe several morning fitness benefits. To mention a few, You'll eat fewer calories; you'll have more energy throughout the day, burn more bothersome fat cells, and sleep better when the sun goes down.

3. She Consumes a Lot of Vegetables.

If you don't pay attention when your mother or your partner softly encourages you to eat more of Mother Earth's natural creations, maybe you'll listen to Oprah Winfrey.

Oprah confessed in an interview that she values her lunch more than any other meal, and one of her meals go-to involves a big, overflowing salad of green goodness. She noted that the salad is usually from the veggies from her home garden. As she put its's "as a rule, if we can grow it, we don't buy it."

You probably don't need us to tell you that veggies are excellent for your diet. Still, science backs up Winfrey's meal plan, as a well-balanced, vegetable patch diet can help fight cancer, heart disease, diabetes, and hypertension, among other conditions.

4. Oprah Schedules Time To Unwind.

There's no doubt that Winfrey's itinerary would be overwhelming for most people, with regular meetings, phone conversations, and traveling, but achieving this degree of esteem necessitates astute management and perseverance. However, if you look into the lives of individuals at the pinnacle of success, such as Winfrey, you'll notice that they constantly make time to unwind.

In an interview about her daily life, Winfrey stated that she relaxes before retiring to bed by reading frequently. Though you may not have Winfrey's gorgeous fireplace to warm you up as you flip the pages over, the research found that individuals who read before bed are less anxious than those who watch Netflix.

5. Practicing Gratitude daily.

The benefits of practicing Gratitude have been proven for centuries, even though gestures to the same have become popular recently. Oprah maintains with her volumes of gratitude diaries that she usually jots down before going to bed. She makes a list of things that have given her tremendous joy or which she is grateful for.

Implementing this habit will not only improve your health but also increase your empathy and self-confidence. One study suggests that thinking about what you're thankful for rather than contemplating on the to-do list each night helps better your sleep.

6. She Manages Her Finances.

You'd think someone of Winfrey's caliber would employ someone to manage her finances, but while she got a whole team, she oversees the minutiae of her fortune daily. She claims that she cannot delegate all financial decisions to others because she had a poor upbringing and prefers to understand what comes in and what goes out of her earnings. She noted during an interview that it is crucial for her to personally manage her finances as doing so relieves her from surprises of what she has and doesn't have.

While most of us struggle with the very thought about money, research has shown that the more you train yourself to handle your finances, the better your chances of becoming wealthy.

Conclusion

Just as Oprah, if you are invariably striving to achieve greatness in all life aspects, you must maintain a couple of healthy habits. If Oprah's journey inspires you, then flexing to the above routine might be your thing. Who knows!

Chapter 30:

How to Reprogram Your Mind for

Success

Your routines are the things that drive you through life. Your routines are driven by your emotions. Your emotions are a sum of your past. Your past is a sum of incidents. These incidents may be related to a person or a thing, which in turn make your life exciting.

You start your day with a thought. A thought that wakes you up every day. A unique thought that everyone experiences every morning. These thoughts are the driving force for you to get up whether you like it or not.

These thoughts may be fear-driven or love memories. So your brain creates emotions in your subconscious mind which in turn dictates your daily tasks and routine.

You might be having doubts about a leave from a job that you might deserve because you can't get the doubt of getting fired out of your mind.

You might be remembering a loved one that you want to see today.

You may be hoping to get some good news today.

So you have a set routine every day, that you follow without even ever pondering on day-to-day life. And this is the ultimate failure of your purpose in life.

A routine that is not getting you forward in life isn't worth living with. But you are not able to think about it because your mind and your subconscious have taken over your body.

As all these obvious things are being stated, close your eyes, put some music on, shut the doors or sit on a bench in a quiet part. Tell your mind to get rid of those memories that drive your emotions. Leave your body motionless and try to take deep breaths.

As you start doing this, you will feel an immediate thought kick in your subconscious. Your mind will be making you feel like something is missing or if you had something to do.

This is an uncomfortable state of mind. But now is your time to be your own master. Tell your subconscious that it is your will that leads you, but not the emotions and your mind.

You have to realize the reality and make it seem more acceptable to your brain. You have to make it feel confident and feel that it is helping you to stay commited in any situation that comes across in your life.

You need to become conscious in this hectic world of involuntary unconsciousness.

You have to make yourself ready for the unpredictable future. Because if you are not ready for the future, you are still drowning in your past.

Everyone's past is toxic. Even good memories can be toxic. One might ask how.

The memories of the past either make your stay in the bed or they make you hope full of chances to come with luck. But luck is rarely lucky.

You cannot be a free man till you dive out of your personal reality that your brain has created to keep you in your comfort zone. You cannot become successful if you stay on your laptop or your phone interacting with the world via social media and emails.

You have to create your own environment by making new friends, taking new jobs, asking questions to your partner, making a change in your natural habitat.

Your mind is the curator of your environment and the people in it. So you have to change your environment by making your mind commit to your orders.

Give your mind a free space to rehabilitate and renew itself. Give it a chance to imagine new things. Make it wander off like a herd of cattle in the grasslands. Let it flow without any emotion, just to create enough space for new realities to pop in. As soon as it does, you will find yourself in a new realm of happiness and success.

Chapter 31:

6 Ways To Adopt New Actions That Will Be Beneficial To Your Life

There is this myth that goes around saying that, once you leave your teenage, you can never change your Habits. One can analyze this for themselves. Everyone has a list of new year's resolutions and goals. We hope to get these things done to some extent, but, never do we ever really have a clear idea of how to get to those goals in the least possible time.

We always desire a better future but never really know how to bring the necessary change in our lives. The change we need is a change in attitude and behavior towards life altogether. Change is never easy, but it is achievable with some sheer willpower. You might be on the right track to lead a better life, but there are always more and better things to add to your daily habits that can be helpful in your daily life.

Here are 6 simple yet achievable actions you need to take:

1. Decide Today What Is Most Important In Your Life

Life is a constant search for motivation. The motivation to keep doing and changing for the better. Once you have something to change for, take a moment and envision the rest of your life with and without the change you are about to make.

If you have made up your mind, now think about how you can start off with these things. For starters, if you want a healthy lifestyle, start your day with a healthy breakfast and morning exercise on an empty stomach. If you want to scale your business, make a customer-friendly business model.

2. Make Reasonable and Achievable Goals.

Adopting new habits can be challenging, especially if you have to change something in your day-to-day life to get better results. Start easy by making goals that are small, easy, reasonable, and won't give you a headache.

You can start off with baby steps. If you want to become more responsible, mature, and sorted in your life, just start your day by making your own bed, and do your dishes. Ride a bicycle to work, instead of a car or a bus. Things become smooth and easier once you have a reason for the hard acts.

3. Erase Distractions from Your Daily Life

You have wasted a lot already, don't waste any more time. As young as you are right now, you should feel more privileged than the older people around you. You have got the luxury of time over them. You have the right energy and pinnacle moments to seize every opportunity you can grasp.

Don't make your life a cluster of meaningless and profit-less distractions. You don't have to go to every public gathering that you are invited to. Only those that give you something in return. Something that you can avail yourself of in your years to come. Don't divulge in these distractions only for the sake of memories. Memories fade but the time you waste will always have its imprint in every moment that follows.

4. Make a Diary and a Music Playlist

You can devote some time to yourself, just to communicate with your brain and start a discussion with yourself. Most people keep a diary for this purpose, some people tend to make a digital one these days. When you start writing to yourself in the third person, talking and discussing your issues and your weaknesses, you tend to find the solutions within.

Most people find it comforting and calming when they have a playlist of music playing in the background while working. Everyone can try this to check if they get a better level of creativity if they have some small activity that soothes their stressed nerves.

5. Incorporate Regular Walk and Exercise in Your Life

When you know you have a whole day ahead of you, where you have to sit in an office chair for the next 8 hours. Where you have to sit in your home office looking at those sheets for most of the day. A 10 min walk before or after the busy schedule can help a lot in such conditions. You can never avoid physical activities for your whole life, especially if you want to live a healthier and longer life.

People always feel reluctant to exercise and running once they enter college or work life. Especially once they have a family to look out for. But trust me, your body needs that blood rushing once a day for some time. You will feel much more pumped and motivated after a hard 2-mile jog or a 15 min workout.

6. Ask Others for Help and Advice

You have a life to live for yourself, but always remember, you are never too old to ask for help. A human can never perfect something in their life. You will always find someone better than you at a particular task, don't shy to ask for help, and never hold back to ask for any advice.

We feel low many a time in our lives. Sometimes we get some foul thoughts, but we shouldn't ever pounce on them. We should rather seek someone's company for comfort and sharing our concerns.

Conclusion

The ultimate success in life is the comfort you get at the end of every day. Life can never be fruitful, beneficial, and worth living for if we don't arrange our lives as resourceful human beings. Productive minds always find a way to counter things and make the best out of everything, and this is the art of living your life.

Chapter 32:

8 Ways To Adopt New Thoughts That Will Be Beneficial To Your Life

"Each morning we are born again. What we do today is what matters most." - Buddha

Is your glass half-empty or half-full? Answering this age-old question may reflect your outlook on life, your attitude toward yourself, whether you're optimistic or pessimistic, or it may even affect your health. Studies show that personality traits such as optimism and pessimism play a considerable role in determining your health and well-being. The positive thinking that comes with optimism is a practical part of stress management. Positive thinking in no way means that we keep our heads in the sand and ignore life's less pleasant situations. Instead, you have to approach the unpleasantness more positively and productively. Always think that something best is going to happen, and ignore the worst-case scenarios.

Here are some ways for you to adopt new thoughts that will benefit your outlook on life.

1. Breaking Out Old Thinking Patterns

We all can get stuck in a loop of specific thoughts. Sure, they may look comfortable on the outside, but we don't realize that these thoughts are what's holding us back most of the time. It's crucial to let fresh ideas and thoughts into your life and break away from the negative ones to see new paths ahead. We could start by challenging our assumptions in every situation. We may already assume what's about to happen if we fall into some condition, but trying new preconceptions can open up some exciting possibilities for us.

2. Rephrase The Problem

Your creativity can get limited by how you define or frame your problems. If you keep on looking at the problem from one side only, chances are you won't get much exposure to the solution. Whereas, if you look at it in different ways and different angles, new solutions can emerge. For example, the founder of Uber, Garret Camp, could have focused on buying and managing enough vehicles for him to make a profit. Instead, he looked more into how he could best entertain the passengers and thus, made a powerful app for their comfort.

3. Think In Reverse

Try turning the problem upside-down if you're having difficulties finding a new approach. Flip the situation and explore the opposite of what you want to achieve. This can help you present innovative ways to tackle the real issue. If you're going to take a good picture, try all of its angles first so you can understand which grade will be more suitable and which angles you should avoid. If you want to develop a new design for your website, try its worst look first and then make it the exact opposite. Apply different types of creativity to tackle your problems.

4. Make New Connections

Another way to generate new ideas and beneficial thoughts is by making unique and unexpected connections. Some of the best ideas click to you by chance, you hear or see something utterly unconnected to the situation you're trying to solve, and an idea has occurred to you almost instantly. For instance, architect Mick Pearce developed a groundbreaking climate-control system by taking the concept from the self-cooling mounds built by termites. You can pick on any set of random words, picture prompts, and objects of interest and then look for the novel association between them and your problem.

5. Finding Fresh Perspectives

Adding extra dynamism to your thinking by taking a step back from your usual standpoint and viewing a problem through "fresh eyes" might be beneficial for you to tackle an issue and give new thoughts. You could also talk to someone with a different perspective, life experience, or cultural background and would be surprised to see their approach. Consider yourself being the other person and see life from their eyes, their point of view.

6. Focus On The Good Things

Challenges and struggles are a part of life. When you're faced with obstacles, try and focus on the good part, no matter how seemingly insignificant or small it seems. If you keep looking for it, you will definitely find the proverbial silver lining in every cloud if it's not evident in the beginning.

7. Practice Gratitude

Practicing gratitude is said to reduce stress, foster resilience, and improve self-esteem. If you're going through a bad time, think of people, moments, or things that bring you some kind of comfort and happiness and express your gratitude once in a while. This could be anything, from thanking your loved one to lending a helping hand to anyone.

8. Practice Positive Self-Talk

We sometimes are our own worst critics and tend to be the hardest on ourselves. This can cause you to form a negative opinion of yourself. This could be prevented by practicing positive self-talk. As a result, this could influence your ability to regulate your feelings, thoughts, and behaviors under stress.

Conclusion

Developing a positive attitude can help you in many ways than you might realize. When you practice positive thinking, you consciously or subconsciously don't allow your mind to entertain any negative thoughts. You will start noticing remarkable changes all around you. By reducing your self-limiting beliefs, you will effectively grow as you have never imagined before. You can change your entire outlook on life by harnessing the power of positive thinking. You will also notice a significant boost in your confidence.

Chapter 33:

Why Are You Working So Hard

Your why,

your reason to get up in the morning,

the reason you act,

really is everything - for without it, there could be nothing.

Your why is the partner of your what,

that is what you want to achieve, your ultimate goal.

Your why will be what pushes you through the hard times on the path to your dreams.

It may be your children or a burning desire to help those less fortunate,

whatever the reason may be,

it is important to keep that in mind when faced with troubles or distractions.

Knowing what you want to do, and why you are doing it,

is of imperative importance for your life.

The tragedy is that most people are aiming for nothing.

They couldn't tell you why they are working in a certain field even if they tried.

Apart from the obvious financial payment,

They have no clue why they are there.

Is financial survival alone really a good motive to act?

Or would financial prosperity be guaranteed if you pursued greater personal preference?

Whatever your ambitions or preference in life,

make sure your why is important enough to you to guarantee your persistence.

Sometimes when pursuing a burning desire,

we can become distracted from the reason we are working.

Your why should be reflected in everything you do.

Once you convince yourself that your reason is important enough, you will not stop.

Despite the hardships, despite the fear, despite the loss and pain.

As long as you maintain a steady path of faith and resilience,

your work will soon start to pay off.

A light will protrude from the darkness and the illusionary troubles sent to test your faith will disappear as if they were never here.

Your why must be strong.

Your what must be as clear as the day is to you now.

And your faith must be eternal and unwavering.

Only then will the doors be opened to you.

This dream can be real, and will be.

When it is clear in the mind with faith, the world will move to show you the way.

The way will be revealed piece by piece, requiring you to take action and do the required work to bring your dream into reality.

Your why is so incredibly important.
The bigger your why, the greater the urgency, and the quicker your action will be.

Take the leap of faith.
Do what you didn't even know you could.
Never mind anyone else.
Taking the unknown path.
Perhaps against the advice of your family and friend,
But you know what your heart wants.

You know that even though the path will be dangerous, the reward will be tremendous.
The risks of not never finding out is too great.
The risk of never knowing if you could have done better is unfathomable.
You can always do better, and you must.

Knowing what is best for you may prove to be the most important thing for you.
How you feel about the work you are doing,
How you feel about the life you are living,
And how do you make the most of the time you have on this earth.
These may prove far more important than financial reward could ever do for you.

Aim to strike a balance.

A balance between working on what you are passionate about and building a wealthy financial life.

If your why and will are strong enough,

Success is all but guaranteed for you – no second guesses needed.

Aim for the sky,

However high you make it,

you will have proven you can indeed fly.

www.ingramcontent.com/pod-product-compliance
Lightning Source LLC
Chambersburg PA
CBHW050743030426
42336CB00012B/1628